I0096712

This publication is intended to provide educational information for the reader on the covered subjects. It is not intended to take the place of personalized medical counseling, diagnosis, and treatment from a trained healthcare professional.

ISBN 978-1-998455-91-1 (Paperback)
ISBN 978-1-998455-92-8 (eBook)

Printed and bound in USA
Published by Loons Press

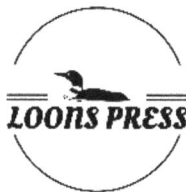

LOONS PRESS

Table Of Contents

How To Prevent Mpox Virus

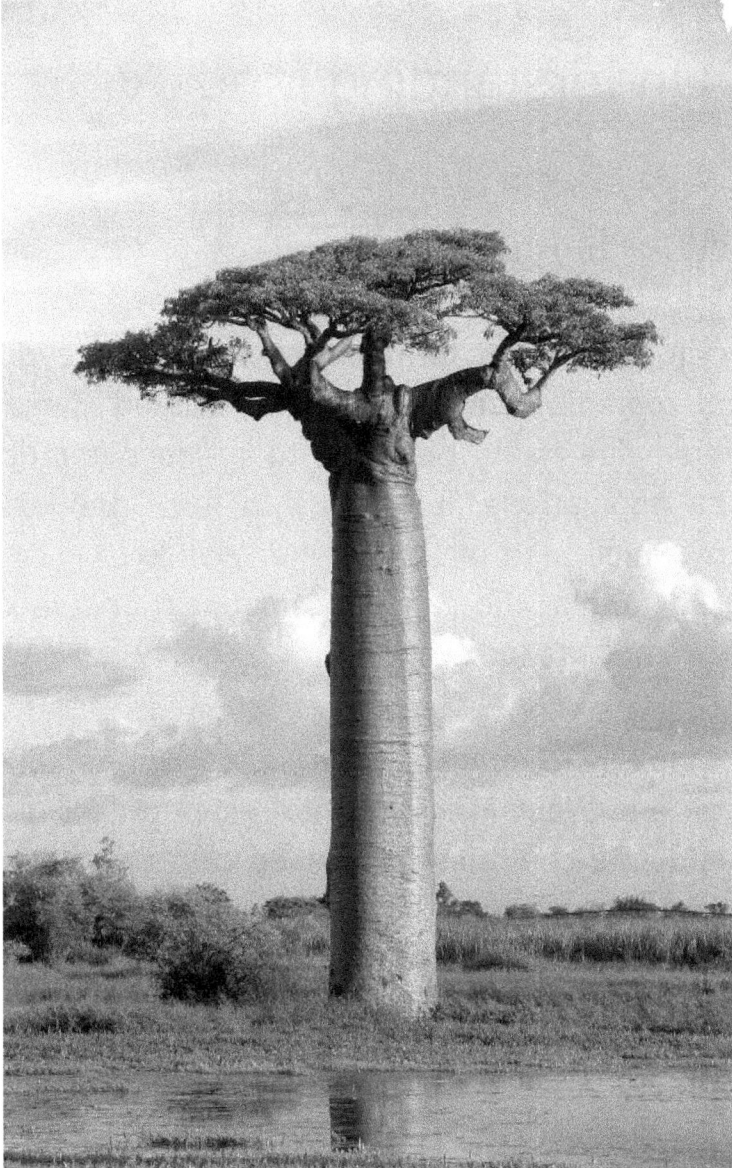

A Comprehensive Guide

Chapter 1

Understanding Mpox Virus

What is Mpox Virus?

The Mpox virus, formerly known as monkeypox, is a viral zoonotic disease that has garnered increasing attention due to its potential to cause outbreaks in human populations. It belongs to the Orthopoxvirus genus, which also includes other well-known viruses such as variola (the cause of smallpox) and vaccinia (used in the smallpox vaccine).

Mpox is primarily found in certain regions of Central and West Africa, but its recent emergence in non-endemic countries has raised concerns about its spread. Understanding the nature of this virus is crucial for effective prevention and response strategies.

Transmission of the Mpox virus can occur through direct contact with infected animals, humans, or surfaces contaminated with the virus. The natural reservoirs for Mpox are believed to be rodents, with primates also being susceptible.

Human-to-human transmission can occur via respiratory droplets during close contact, or through bodily fluids and skin lesions. The virus has an incubation period of approximately 7 to 14 days, though it can range from 5 to 21 days. Symptoms typically begin with fever, headache, muscle aches, and fatigue, followed by the development of a distinctive rash that progresses through various stages.

The clinical presentation of Mpox can often be mistaken for other illnesses, such as chickenpox or measles, making accurate diagnosis imperative. The rash usually starts on the face before spreading to other parts of the body, and its progression through stages—macules, papules, vesicles, pustules, and scabs—can help differentiate it from other viral infections.

The disease can vary in severity, with some individuals experiencing mild symptoms while others face more serious complications, particularly in those with weakened immune systems.

Given the potential for outbreaks and the serious health implications associated with Mpox, awareness and prevention strategies are essential. Public health measures focus on educating communities about the risks of the virus and the importance of avoiding contact with potentially infected animals or individuals.

Vaccination remains one of the most effective tools for prevention, especially for at-risk populations. The smallpox vaccine has shown cross-protective effects against Mpox, and health authorities may recommend it in response to outbreaks.

In conclusion, understanding the Mpox virus is vital for anyone concerned about its impact on public health. By learning about its transmission, symptoms, and prevention measures, individuals can take proactive steps to protect themselves and their communities.

As research continues to evolve, staying informed about the Mpox virus will be key to mitigating its effects and ensuring a swift public health response to any future outbreaks.

History and Outbreaks

The history of the Mpox virus, previously known as monkeypox, traces its origins back to the late 1950s when it was first identified in laboratory monkeys in Denmark. However, it is believed that the virus is endemic to certain regions of Central and West Africa, where it was initially transmitted to humans through contact with infected animals.

The first recorded human case was documented in 1970 in the Democratic Republic of the Congo. Since then, the Mpox virus has been associated with sporadic outbreaks, primarily in rural areas where people may come into close contact with infected wildlife, such as rodents and primates.

Over the years, several outbreaks of Mpox have been reported, with varying degrees of severity. The most significant outbreak occurred in the Democratic Republic of the Congo during the late 1990s and early 2000s, where the incidence rate soared. This alarming increase highlighted the need for enhanced surveillance and public health measures in affected regions. Other notable outbreaks occurred outside of Africa, particularly in the United States in 2003, when a cluster of cases was linked to pet prairie dogs that had been imported from Africa, demonstrating the virus's potential to spread beyond its endemic areas.

The Mpox virus can manifest with symptoms similar to those of smallpox, including fever, rash, and swollen lymph nodes. While the disease generally has a lower mortality rate compared to smallpox, it poses significant health risks, especially among immunocompromised individuals and children. The outbreaks have prompted public health authorities to implement quarantine measures and vaccination campaigns aimed at controlling the spread. The re-emergence of Mpox has raised concerns about zoonotic diseases and their potential impact on public health, emphasizing the need for continued vigilance.

How To Prevent Mpox Virus

In recent years, there has been a resurgence of Mpox cases, particularly in non-endemic countries. The increased global travel and trade in wildlife have facilitated the spread of the virus, prompting health organizations to re-evaluate their preparedness strategies. The World Health Organization (WHO) and the Centers for Disease Control and Prevention (CDC) have emphasized the importance of awareness and education on Mpox, particularly in communities that may be at higher risk. Public health campaigns focusing on the transmission routes, symptoms, and preventive measures are crucial in controlling potential outbreaks.

Understanding the history and patterns of Mpox outbreaks is essential for effective prevention strategies. It highlights the ongoing risk of zoonotic diseases and the importance of proactive measures to mitigate the spread of the virus. Individuals concerned about Mpox should stay informed about the latest developments and adhere to recommended guidelines to protect themselves and their communities. By fostering awareness and promoting preventive actions, we can collectively work towards minimizing the impact of Mpox and safeguarding public health.

Symptoms and Transmission

Understanding the symptoms and transmission of the Mpox virus is crucial for effective prevention. The initial symptoms typically manifest within one to three weeks after exposure to the virus. Individuals may experience fever, headache, muscle aches, backache, swollen lymph nodes, chills, and fatigue.

One of the hallmark signs of Mpox is the development of a rash, which can appear on the face and body, often following the fever. This rash can progress through stages, starting as flat lesions that become raised, filled with fluid, and eventually crust over. Recognizing these symptoms early can be instrumental in seeking timely medical attention and reducing the spread of the virus.

Transmission of the Mpox virus primarily occurs through direct contact with the lesions, bodily fluids, or respiratory droplets from an infected person. The virus can also be transmitted through contact with contaminated materials, such as clothing or bedding, that have been used by an infected individual.

While respiratory transmission is possible, it requires prolonged face-to-face interaction, making it less common in casual encounters. Understanding these transmission routes is essential for individuals to take appropriate precautions, especially in settings where close contact is common.

In addition to human-to-human transmission, Mpox can also spread through zoonotic means. Certain animals, particularly rodents and primates, can harbor the virus and transmit it to humans. Engaging in activities that involve handling or coming into contact with these animals, particularly in areas where Mpox is endemic, poses a risk. Thus, awareness of one's environment and potential exposure sources is a vital preventive measure to mitigate the risk of infection.

Preventing transmission of the Mpox virus involves implementing basic hygiene practices and awareness of exposure risks. Regular handwashing with soap and water, or using hand sanitizer when soap is unavailable, can significantly reduce the likelihood of virus spread.

Additionally, individuals should avoid close contact with anyone exhibiting symptoms of Mpox, particularly those with visible skin lesions. If a person is diagnosed with the virus, they should follow public health guidelines regarding isolation and inform close contacts about their potential exposure.

Overall, being informed about the symptoms and transmission of the Mpox virus is a key component in the fight against its spread. By recognizing the early signs of infection and understanding how the virus can be transmitted, individuals can take proactive steps to protect themselves and others. Education and awareness are powerful tools in preventing Mpox, allowing communities to respond effectively and reduce the impact of this viral infection.

How To Prevent Mpox Virus

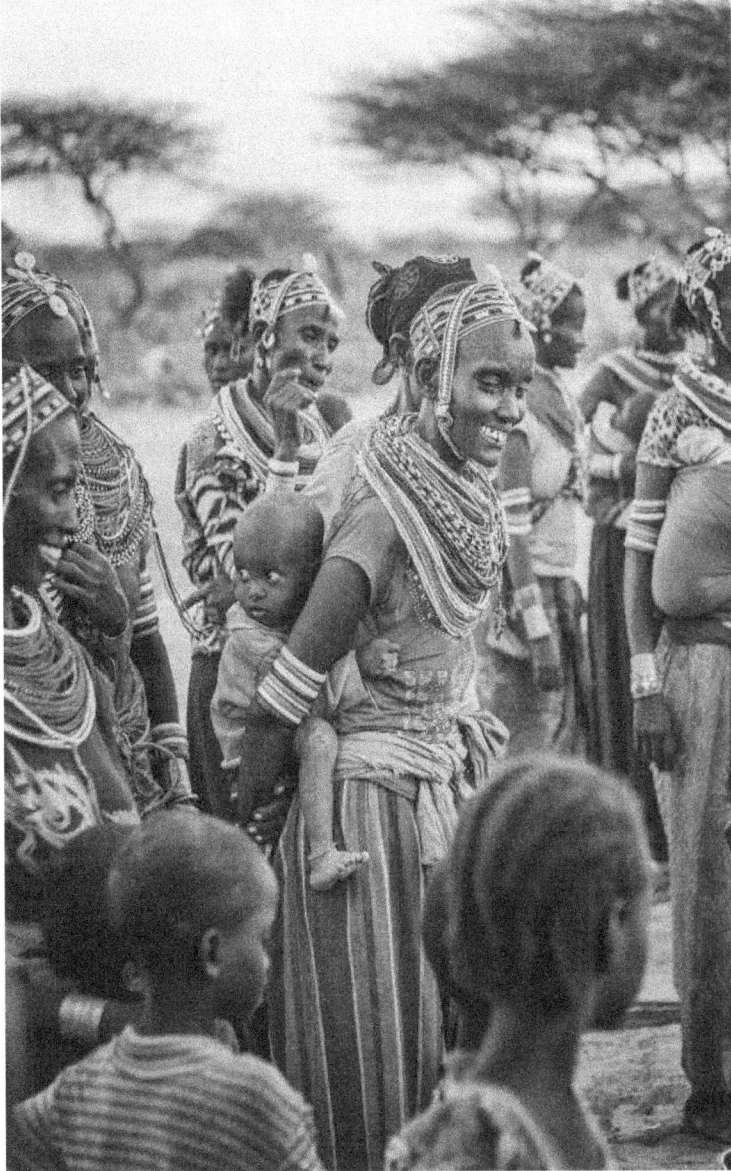

Chapter 2

Risk Factors

Who is at Risk?

In the context of the Mpox virus, understanding who is at risk is crucial for effective prevention and protection strategies. Mpox primarily spreads through close contact with infected individuals, making certain population groups more vulnerable. This risk is heightened in environments where close physical interactions occur, such as households, healthcare settings, and communities with reduced access to healthcare resources. Awareness of these risk factors can empower individuals and communities to take proactive measures in safeguarding their health.

One of the primary groups at risk includes individuals who engage in close physical contact, particularly in social or sexual settings. This group often includes men who have sex with men, as studies have shown a higher incidence of Mpox cases among this population.

However, it is essential to recognize that anyone with close contact to an infected person can contract the virus, regardless of sexual orientation or lifestyle. This underscores the importance of comprehensive education on transmission risks and safe practices for all individuals.

Healthcare workers face significant risks as well, especially those who may come into contact with infected patients without proper personal protective equipment (PPE). Inadequate training or resources can lead to increased exposure, making it vital for healthcare facilities to implement strict infection control protocols. Training staff on recognizing symptoms and understanding transmission dynamics can mitigate risks and protect both healthcare providers and patients from potential outbreaks.

Moreover, individuals with compromised immune systems are at an elevated risk of severe illness if infected with the Mpox virus. This includes patients with chronic diseases, those undergoing immunosuppressive treatments, and individuals living with HIV/AIDS.

For these populations, prevention strategies must be prioritized, including vaccination where available, education on recognizing early symptoms, and guidance on avoiding high-risk situations. Tailoring prevention efforts to meet the specific needs of these vulnerable groups is key to reducing overall transmission rates.

Finally, it is essential to consider the role of misinformation and stigma in perpetuating the spread of Mpox. Communities often bear the brunt of social stigma, which can discourage individuals from seeking care or reporting symptoms. This creates a cycle of risk that can lead to larger outbreaks.

Public health campaigns must focus on dispelling myths surrounding the virus, promoting a message of inclusivity, and encouraging everyone to engage in safe behaviors. By fostering an informed and supportive community, we can collectively enhance our resilience against the Mpox virus and protect those most at risk.

High-Risk Behaviors

High-risk behaviors play a significant role in the transmission of the Mpox virus, a disease that has gained attention in recent years due to its potential to spread in certain populations. Understanding these behaviors is crucial for individuals who are concerned about preventing the virus.

This subchapter will explore the various high-risk activities associated with Mpox transmission and provide practical recommendations for minimizing exposure.

One of the most notable high-risk behaviors involves close physical contact with infected individuals. Mpox is primarily transmitted through direct contact with the lesions, bodily fluids, or respiratory droplets of an infected person. Engaging in intimate activities, such as sexual intercourse or sharing bedding, can significantly increase the risk of exposure. To reduce this risk, it is essential to avoid close contact with anyone exhibiting symptoms of Mpox, including rashes or lesions that resemble those associated with the disease.

Another critical area of concern is travel to regions experiencing Mpox outbreaks. Individuals traveling to areas where the virus is prevalent may inadvertently engage in high-risk behaviors due to a lack of awareness or information about the local health situation. It is advisable for travelers to stay informed about health advisories and potential outbreaks in their destination. Practicing good hygiene, such as frequent handwashing and avoiding crowded places, can help mitigate the risk of contracting the virus while traveling.

Participation in large gatherings or events can also pose a heightened risk for Mpox transmission. Crowded environments create opportunities for close contact with others, increasing the likelihood of exposure to respiratory droplets or skin contact with individuals who may be infected.

To protect oneself and others, it is important to consider the safety measures in place at such events. Opting for outdoor gatherings, maintaining physical distance, and wearing masks can significantly reduce the chances of virus transmission in these settings.

Finally, the sharing of personal items, such as clothing or towels, can facilitate the spread of the Mpox virus. Items that come into contact with an infected person's skin or bodily fluids can harbor the virus and transmit it to others. To minimize this risk, individuals should avoid sharing personal belongings and ensure that items are properly sanitized.

Additionally, practicing good hygiene, such as washing hands frequently and using hand sanitizer, can further decrease the likelihood of transmission through indirect contact.

In summary, recognizing and addressing high-risk behaviors is essential in the fight against the Mpox virus. By avoiding close contact with infected individuals, staying informed while traveling, being cautious in crowded environments, and practicing good hygiene, individuals can significantly reduce their risk of exposure. Awareness and proactive measures are key components in preventing Mpox and protecting both personal health and public safety.

Environmental Factors

Understanding the environmental factors that contribute to the spread of the Mpox virus is crucial for effective prevention. The Mpox virus, like many other infectious agents, can thrive in specific conditions that facilitate its transmission. These factors include temperature, humidity, and the presence of suitable hosts. By recognizing and mitigating these environmental influences, individuals can better safeguard themselves and their communities against the virus.

Temperature plays a significant role in the survival and transmission of the Mpox virus. Research indicates that the virus remains viable for varying periods depending on environmental temperatures. Warmer temperatures can accelerate the decay of the virus on surfaces, while cooler conditions may prolong its lifespan. This means that in regions experiencing fluctuating weather patterns, the risk of transmission can change rapidly. Individuals should be aware of their local climate and adjust their preventive measures accordingly, particularly during colder months when viral persistence may be higher.

Humidity is another critical factor that influences the Mpox virus's viability. High humidity levels can create a conducive environment for the virus, as moisture can help it survive on surfaces longer. Conversely, very low humidity can lead to the desiccation of the virus, reducing its infectivity.

Communities in humid climates should prioritize frequent cleaning and disinfection of shared surfaces, especially in public places such as schools, healthcare facilities, and public transportation. Utilizing air conditioning and dehumidifiers can also help maintain indoor humidity levels that are less favorable for the virus.

The presence of suitable hosts in the environment significantly impacts the transmission dynamics of the Mpox virus. Animals play a pivotal role in the ecology of this virus, acting as reservoirs and contributing to outbreaks. Understanding the wildlife and domestic animal populations in a given area can inform preventive strategies. For instance, avoiding contact with potentially infected animals and ensuring that pets are kept indoors can reduce the risk of zoonotic transmission.

Additionally, community education on recognizing and reporting unusual animal behavior can help in early detection and response to potential outbreaks.

Lastly, the built environment, including urban planning and public health infrastructure, can influence the spread of the Mpox virus. Areas with high population density may facilitate faster transmission due to close contact among individuals. Improving sanitation, waste management, and public health resources can mitigate these risks. Individuals should advocate for community-level initiatives that enhance environmental conditions, such as better waste disposal systems and public health campaigns focused on hygiene practices. By addressing these environmental factors collectively, communities can create safer spaces that reduce the likelihood of Mpox virus transmission.

How To Prevent Mpox Virus

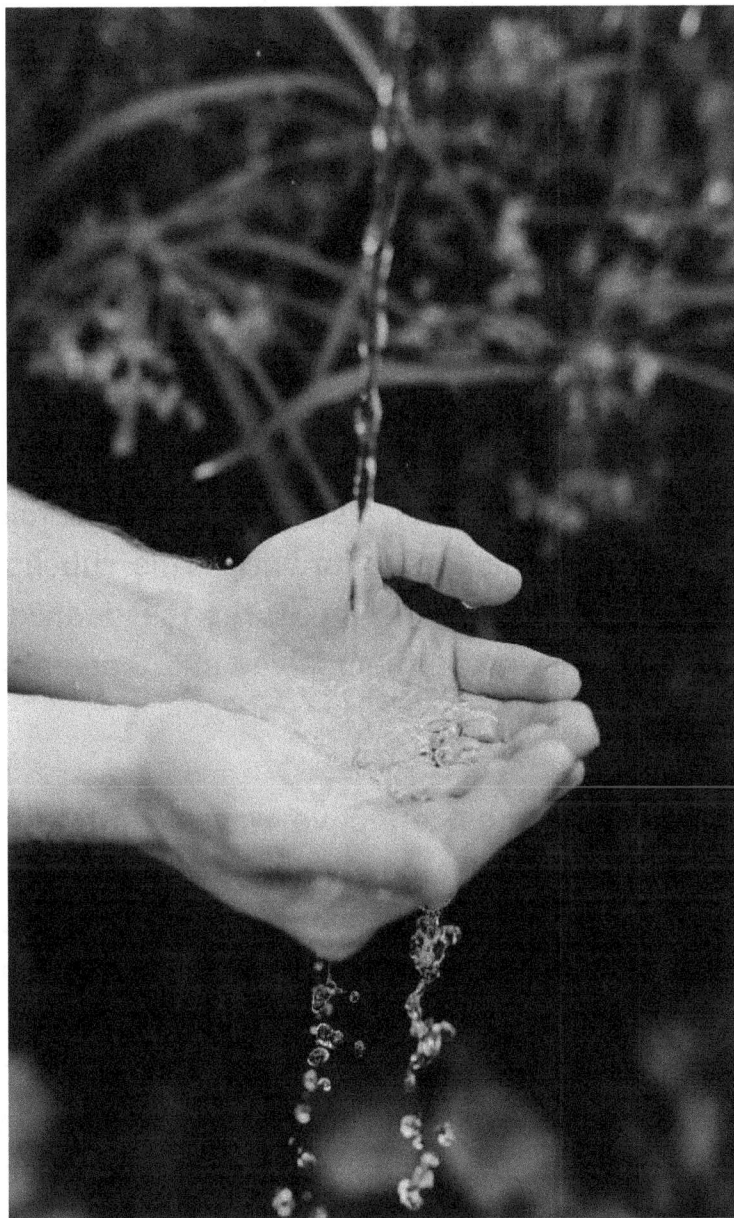

Chapter 3

Preventive Measures

Personal Hygiene Practices

Maintaining personal hygiene is a foundational element in preventing the spread of the Mpox virus. Proper hygiene practices not only reduce the risk of contracting the virus but also play a crucial role in protecting others in the community. This subchapter outlines essential hygiene measures that individuals can adopt to safeguard themselves and those around them.

One of the most effective ways to prevent the transmission of the Mpox virus is through regular handwashing. Individuals should wash their hands thoroughly with soap and water for at least 20 seconds, especially after being in public spaces, using the restroom, or before eating. In situations where soap and water are not available, using a hand sanitizer that contains at least 60% alcohol can serve as an effective alternative.

It is important to ensure that all surfaces of the hands, including between the fingers and under the nails, are cleaned to eliminate any potential viral particles.

In addition to hand hygiene, it is crucial to maintain cleanliness in personal items and shared surfaces. Regularly disinfecting frequently touched surfaces such as doorknobs, light switches, and mobile devices can significantly reduce the likelihood of viral transmission. Using disinfectants that are effective against viruses, as recommended by health authorities, is essential. Individuals should also be mindful of their personal items, such as towels and razors, and avoid sharing these with others to minimize the risk of cross-contamination.

The importance of personal grooming cannot be overstated in the context of Mpox virus prevention. Regular bathing and the use of clean clothing can help eliminate any potential viral presence on the skin. Individuals should also ensure that any cuts or abrasions are properly cleaned and covered to prevent infection. Maintaining a clean and healthy appearance not only contributes to personal well-being but also promotes a culture of health in the community.

Lastly, it is essential to stay informed about best practices for personal hygiene in relation to Mpox virus prevention. This includes being aware of any updates or recommendations from health organizations regarding hygiene measures. Engaging in community education about the significance of personal hygiene can further enhance collective efforts to reduce the spread of the virus. By adopting and promoting strong personal hygiene practices, individuals can play a vital role in the fight against the Mpox virus and contribute to a healthier society.

Safe Encounters and Interactions

Safe Encounters and Interactions are crucial aspects of preventing the spread of the Mpox virus. As communities continue to navigate the challenges posed by this virus, understanding how to engage safely with others is paramount. The Mpox virus, primarily transmitted through close contact, necessitates a proactive approach to interactions, whether in social settings, workplaces, or even within families. By adopting safe practices, individuals can significantly reduce their risk of exposure while fostering a sense of community and care.

First and foremost, it is essential to recognize the importance of physical distancing. Maintaining a safe distance from others, especially in crowded or enclosed spaces, minimizes the likelihood of transmission. This is particularly relevant during gatherings or events where individuals may be in close proximity.

Organizers and attendees alike should promote and adhere to guidelines that encourage spacing, such as arranging seating to allow for distance and limiting the number of participants. Additionally, outdoor gatherings are preferable, as open-air environments reduce the risk of airborne transmission significantly.

Personal hygiene practices play a pivotal role in safe encounters. Regular handwashing with soap and water is one of the most effective ways to eliminate potential virus particles that may be present on the hands. When soap and water are unavailable, the use of hand sanitizer containing at least 60% alcohol is recommended.

It is equally important to avoid touching the face, particularly the eyes, nose, and mouth, as this can facilitate the virus's entry into the body. Individuals should also be encouraged to refrain from sharing personal items, such as utensils, drinks, or towels, to further mitigate the risk of transmission during social interactions.

In addition to hygiene and distancing, the use of protective gear should be considered in high-risk situations. Masks can serve as a barrier, particularly in indoor settings or when physical distancing is challenging. Encouraging the use of masks during interactions can drastically reduce the chances of airborne transmission.

Furthermore, staying informed about vaccination and prophylactic measures is vital. Individuals should discuss vaccination options with healthcare providers and understand the benefits of being vaccinated, which can lead to greater community immunity and reduced virus spread.

Finally, fostering open communication about health and safety is essential in any interaction. Individuals should feel empowered to discuss their health status, vaccination status, or any concerns they may have regarding Mpox. Encouraging a culture of transparency can help mitigate fear and stigma associated with the virus, creating a supportive environment where everyone can engage safely.

By prioritizing safe encounters and interactions, communities can work together to protect their members while promoting health and well-being in the face of the Mpox virus.

Travel Safety Tips

Traveling can introduce new risks, especially for individuals concerned about contracting the Mpox virus. As a precaution, it is crucial to be aware of best practices that can minimize exposure and ensure a safer journey. This subchapter outlines essential travel safety tips tailored for those who prioritize their health and well-being while navigating the complexities of travel in a world where infectious diseases can pose a threat.

Before embarking on any trip, research your destination to understand the current Mpox situation. Check the latest health advisories issued by reputable sources such as the Centers for Disease Control and Prevention (CDC) or the World Health Organization (WHO). Understanding the prevalence of Mpox in your destination will help you make informed decisions about your travel plans, including whether to postpone or alter your itinerary based on risk levels.

Additionally, familiarize yourself with local health care facilities, should you need medical assistance while away from home.

Vaccination is one of the most effective ways to protect yourself against Mpox. If you are planning to travel to areas where the virus is prevalent, consult your healthcare provider about getting vaccinated before your trip. While vaccines significantly reduce the risk of infection, they are not 100% effective. Therefore, it is advisable to maintain other preventive measures, such as practicing good hygiene, wearing masks in crowded places, and avoiding close contact with individuals who exhibit symptoms of the virus.

When traveling, prioritize personal hygiene to reduce the risk of Mpox transmission. Regularly washing your hands with soap and water is crucial, especially after touching surfaces in public spaces. If soap and water are not available, use hand sanitizer with at least 60% alcohol content. Avoid touching your face, particularly your eyes, nose, and mouth, as these areas can serve as entry points for viruses. Carry disinfectant wipes to clean surfaces such as airplane trays, hotel room handles, and other frequently touched areas to further decrease the likelihood of infection.

Lastly, consider your social interactions while traveling. Limit close contact with individuals who may exhibit symptoms of Mpox, such as lesions or rashes. Engage with people in open, well-ventilated spaces when possible, and maintain physical distance from crowds. If you find yourself in a situation where you feel unwell or notice any symptoms, seek medical attention promptly and follow local health guidelines. By adhering to these travel safety tips, you can significantly reduce your risk of contracting the Mpox virus and enjoy a safer travel experience.

How To Prevent Mpox Virus

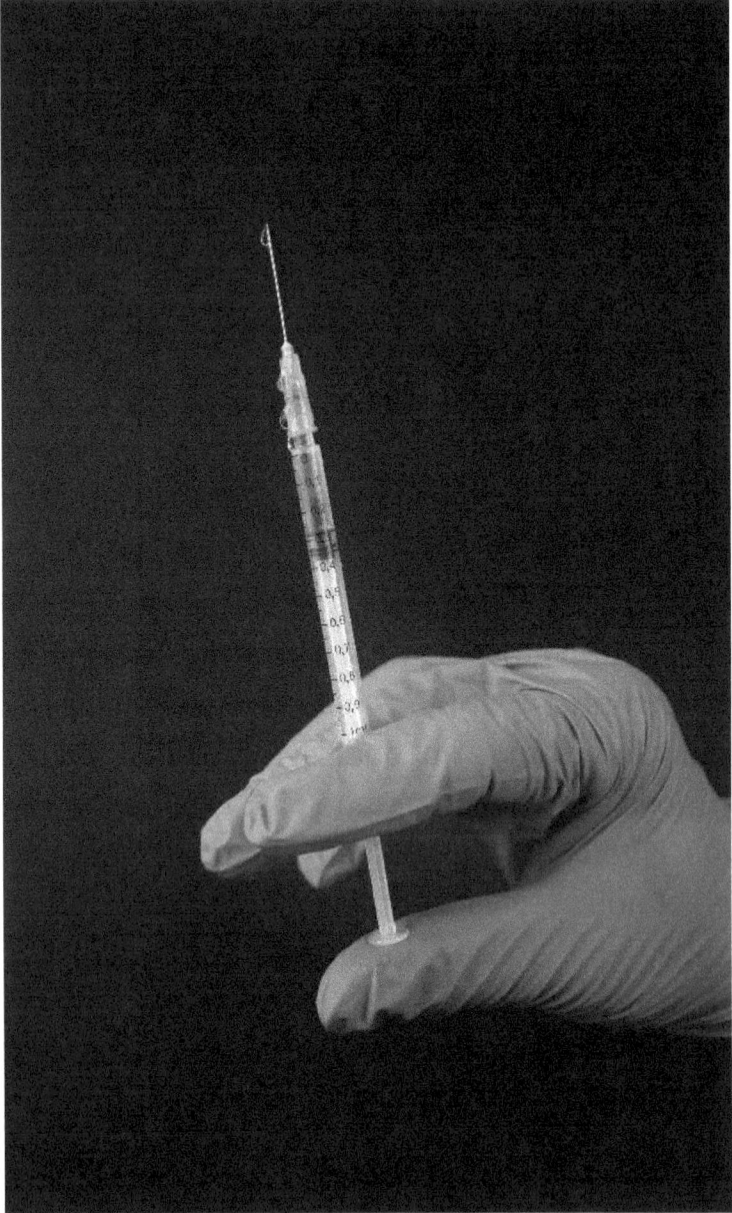

Chapter 4

Vaccination and Treatment

Availability of Vaccines

The availability of vaccines is a crucial aspect of public health strategies aimed at controlling the spread of the Mpox virus. Vaccination not only protects individuals from infection but also contributes to community immunity, reducing overall transmission rates. Understanding the current landscape of vaccine availability is essential for those concerned about Mpox, as it empowers individuals to make informed decisions regarding their health and safety.

Currently, vaccines specifically targeting the Mpox virus are being developed and distributed in various regions. Health authorities around the world have recognized the need for rapid vaccine deployment, especially in areas experiencing outbreaks.

Countries with existing vaccination programs against similar viruses, such as smallpox, have leveraged these frameworks to facilitate the distribution of Mpox vaccines to at-risk populations. This proactive approach aims to curb the transmission of the virus before it escalates into a larger public health crisis.

Access to Mpox vaccines varies significantly across different geographic locations. In some regions, vaccines are readily available at community health centers, clinics, and hospitals, while in others, accessibility may be limited due to logistical challenges or funding constraints.

Public health campaigns play a vital role in raising awareness about the availability of these vaccines and encouraging eligible individuals to get vaccinated. For those concerned about Mpox, staying informed about local vaccination sites and eligibility criteria is a critical step in prevention efforts.

How To Prevent Mpox Virus

It is also important to consider the guidance provided by health organizations regarding who should receive the vaccine. Typically, priority is given to individuals in high-risk categories, such as healthcare workers, individuals with high exposure risk, and certain vulnerable populations. Public health authorities continuously evaluate the situation and may expand eligibility as more vaccines become available or as the epidemiological landscape changes. Understanding these guidelines helps individuals determine their own risk levels and take appropriate actions to protect themselves.

In conclusion, the availability of vaccines against the Mpox virus is an essential element in the fight against this disease. Staying informed about vaccine distribution, eligibility, and local health resources equips individuals with the knowledge they need to safeguard their health and that of their communities.

As the landscape of vaccine availability continues to evolve, ongoing engagement with public health initiatives will remain critical for effectively preventing the spread of Mpox virus and ensuring the well-being of at-risk populations.

Efficacy of Vaccination

Vaccination has emerged as a cornerstone in the fight against infectious diseases, including the Mpox virus. Understanding the efficacy of vaccination is crucial for individuals concerned about their health and the well-being of their communities. Vaccines function by stimulating the immune system to recognize and combat pathogens without causing the disease itself. This process equips the body with the tools needed to fend off future infections, thereby significantly reducing the risk of severe disease, hospitalization, and transmission.

The primary goal of Mpox vaccination is to provide protection against the virus while contributing to herd immunity. When a significant portion of the population is vaccinated, the overall circulation of the virus decreases, making it less likely for unvaccinated individuals to contract the disease. This is particularly important for those who cannot be vaccinated due to health reasons, as it offers them a layer of protection through reduced exposure. Studies have demonstrated that vaccination not only lowers the incidence of Mpox but also mitigates the severity of the illness in those who may still become infected.

How To Prevent Mpox Virus

Research has shown that vaccines targeting the Mpox virus demonstrate a high efficacy rate. Clinical trials and post-marketing studies indicate that vaccinated individuals have a significantly lower risk of contracting the virus compared to those who are unvaccinated. Furthermore, in cases where vaccinated individuals do contract Mpox, the symptoms tend to be milder and of shorter duration. This reduced severity is crucial in preventing complications and the likelihood of transmission to others, reinforcing the importance of widespread vaccination efforts.

Public health initiatives have emphasized the importance of completing the vaccination series to achieve maximum protection. Booster doses may also play a critical role in maintaining immunity over time, especially as the virus evolves.

It is essential for individuals to stay informed about their vaccination status and adhere to recommended schedules. Engaging with healthcare providers can help clarify any concerns regarding the vaccine and ensure that individuals are up to date with their immunizations, contributing to their personal safety and community health.

In conclusion, the efficacy of vaccination against the Mpox virus is a vital component of preventive health strategies. By understanding how vaccines work and their role in reducing both individual and community risk, individuals can make informed decisions about their health. Emphasizing the importance of vaccines can help build a resilient public health infrastructure, ultimately leading to the containment and potential eradication of the Mpox virus. Staying vigilant and proactive in the face of infectious diseases is key to safeguarding both personal and public health.

Treatment Options

The Mpox virus, previously known as monkeypox, has raised significant public health concerns due to its potential for outbreaks and transmission. Understanding the treatment options available is essential for individuals who wish to stay informed and safe. Treatment approaches for Mpox focus on alleviating symptoms, preventing complications, and reducing the risk of transmission. While there is no specific antiviral treatment approved solely for Mpox, several strategies can be employed to manage the disease effectively.

One of the primary treatment options for Mpox is supportive care, which involves addressing the symptoms and complications that arise during infection. This includes managing fever, pain, and skin lesions. Healthcare providers may recommend over-the-counter medications such as acetaminophen or ibuprofen to reduce fever and alleviate discomfort. Maintaining hydration and nutrition is also crucial, as these factors support the immune system in fighting off the virus. Patients are encouraged to rest and monitor their symptoms closely, seeking medical attention if complications arise.

In certain cases, antiviral medications that are effective against similar viruses may be considered as part of the treatment plan. For example, tecovirimat (TPOXX) has been used in treating orthopoxvirus infections and may be administered in severe cases of Mpox, especially for individuals at high risk of complications. The use of such antivirals is typically reserved for those with severe symptoms or for individuals who are immunocompromised. Early intervention with these medications can help reduce the severity of the disease and shorten the duration of symptoms.

Vaccination also plays a critical role in preventing the spread of Mpox and reducing the severity of illness in those who contract the virus. The JYNNEOS vaccine, which is a live virus vaccine, has shown promise in providing immunity against Mpox. It is recommended for individuals who are at increased risk of exposure, including healthcare workers and those in close contact with infected individuals. Receiving the vaccine before exposure can significantly mitigate the risk of contracting the virus or experiencing serious complications if infected.

Lastly, education and awareness are vital components of managing Mpox outbreaks. Individuals should be informed about the symptoms, modes of transmission, and preventive measures to reduce the risk of infection. Public health authorities often provide guidelines and updates regarding vaccination campaigns and treatment options available in the community. By staying informed and proactive, individuals can not only protect themselves but also contribute to the broader effort to control the spread of Mpox. Understanding treatment options empowers concerned citizens to make informed decisions regarding their health and that of their community.

How To Prevent Mpox Virus

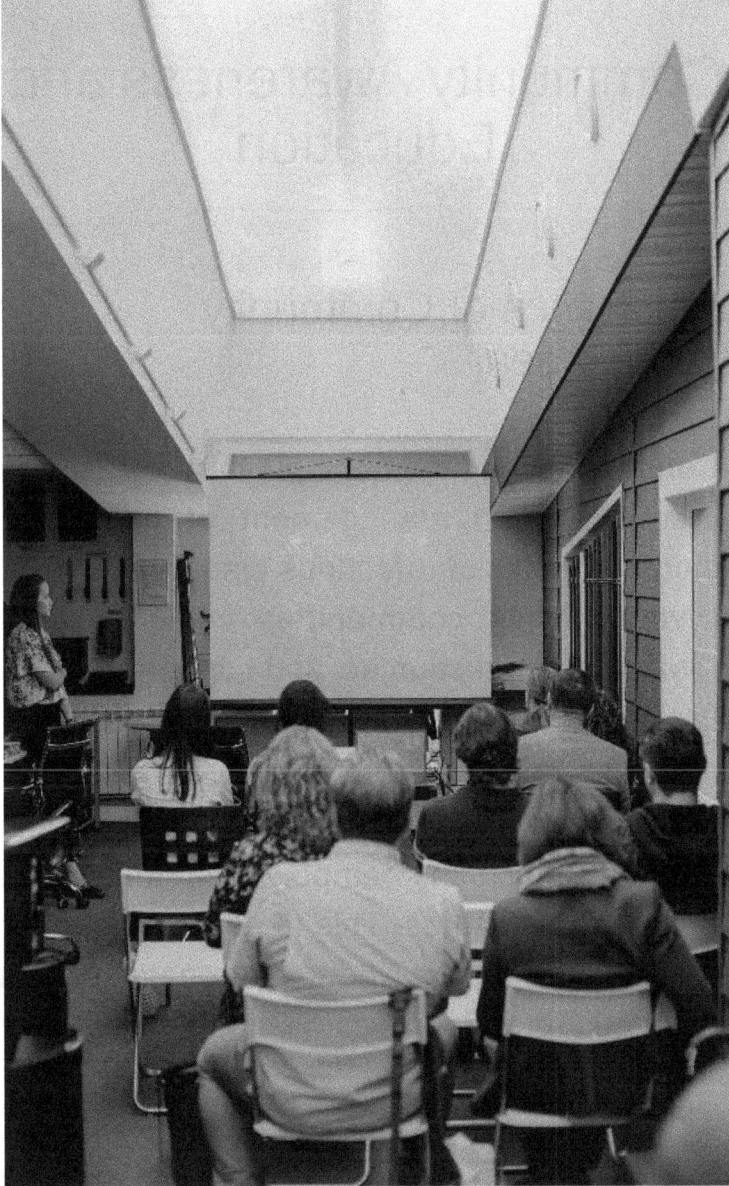

Chapter 5

Community Awareness and Education

Importance of Community Engagement

Community engagement plays a critical role in the prevention and management of health crises, including outbreaks of infectious diseases such as the Mpox virus. When communities come together to share information, resources, and support, they create a robust defense against the spread of illness.

Engaging community members fosters a sense of collective responsibility, empowering individuals to take proactive measures. This is especially important in the context of Mpox, where awareness, education, and shared practices can significantly reduce transmission rates.

How To Prevent Mpox Virus

One of the primary benefits of community engagement is the dissemination of accurate information. Misinformation about Mpox can lead to fear, stigma, and misguided behaviors that exacerbate the situation. By engaging with local health organizations, community leaders, and public health officials, individuals can access reliable resources that clarify the nature of the virus, its modes of transmission, and effective prevention strategies. This shared knowledge equips community members to make informed decisions about their health and the health of those around them.

Community engagement also cultivates a supportive environment that encourages individuals to adopt safe practices. When people see their peers actively participating in preventive measures—such as vaccination, hygiene practices, and awareness campaigns—they are more likely to follow suit. Initiatives like community workshops, informational sessions, and outreach programs can help instill a culture of safety and vigilance. This collective effort can lead to higher vaccination rates and increased compliance with public health recommendations, ultimately lowering the risk of an Mpox outbreak.

Moreover, engaging the community fosters collaboration among various stakeholders, including healthcare providers, local governments, and nonprofit organizations. This collaboration is essential for developing tailored interventions that address specific community needs. For instance, a community with a high prevalence of Mpox may require targeted outreach efforts to reach vulnerable populations.

By working together, these stakeholders can identify gaps in resources and information, ensuring that all segments of the population are informed and protected.

Lastly, community engagement creates a sense of resilience and preparedness. When communities are actively involved in health initiatives, they are better equipped to respond to outbreaks. This preparedness includes having emergency plans, access to necessary resources, and established communication channels.

A community that understands the importance of collaboration and proactive measures can swiftly mobilize when faced with health threats, thus minimizing the potential impact of the Mpox virus. In conclusion, fostering community engagement is not only essential for preventing Mpox but also for cultivating a healthier environment for all.

Educational Resources

In the fight against the Mpox virus, access to reliable educational resources is essential for individuals seeking to mitigate risks and enhance their understanding of the virus. Numerous organizations and health agencies provide comprehensive information that can empower individuals to make informed decisions regarding their health and safety.

These resources range from online platforms to community programs, each offering valuable insights into Mpox prevention strategies, symptoms, transmission modes, and vaccination options.

One of the primary sources of information is the Centers for Disease Control and Prevention (CDC), which offers a wealth of data regarding Mpox. Their website includes detailed guidelines on the virus's epidemiology, preventive measures, and updates on outbreaks. The CDC also produces educational materials, such as brochures and infographics, that break down complex information into digestible formats, making it easier for the public to understand how to protect themselves and their communities.

Additionally, the CDC regularly hosts webinars and training sessions that delve deeper into specific aspects of Mpox prevention, providing an interactive platform for learning.

Local health departments serve as another vital resource for community members. They often conduct outreach programs aimed at educating residents about Mpox and the importance of vaccination and preventive practices. These programs may include public health campaigns, workshops, and informational sessions tailored to specific populations at risk.

Engaging with local health authorities can help individuals stay informed about the latest developments in Mpox prevention and receive guidance on how to access testing and vaccination services.

In addition to governmental resources, various non-profit organizations focus on educating the public about Mpox. These organizations often provide resources tailored to specific communities, including those disproportionately affected by the virus. They may offer support groups, educational materials in multiple languages, and online forums where individuals can share experiences and ask questions. Collaborating with these organizations can enhance community awareness and foster a collective effort to reduce the spread of Mpox, making education a communal responsibility.

Lastly, leveraging social media and online platforms can significantly enhance awareness and access to information about Mpox. Social media campaigns facilitated by health organizations can disseminate crucial information rapidly, reaching a broader audience.

However, it is important to verify the credibility of the sources shared on these platforms, as misinformation can lead to confusion and complacency. By following reputable health organizations and experts, individuals can receive timely updates and educational resources that will aid in understanding and preventing the Mpox virus effectively. Engaging with these educational resources is a proactive step towards ensuring personal and community health in the face of this virus.

Hosting Awareness Campaigns

Hosting awareness campaigns is a crucial strategy in the fight against the Mpox virus. These campaigns serve to educate the public about the virus, its transmission, and the measures that can be taken to prevent infection.

By increasing awareness, communities can empower individuals with the knowledge needed to protect themselves and others. This proactive approach not only helps to dispel myths and misinformation surrounding the virus but also fosters a supportive environment where individuals feel encouraged to engage in preventive practices.

One effective way to host an awareness campaign is through community workshops and seminars. These events can be organized in collaboration with local health departments, educational institutions, and non-profit organizations. Tailoring the content of these workshops to address the specific concerns of the community can enhance engagement and participation. Providing attendees with accurate information about the Mpox virus, including its symptoms and transmission routes, can equip them with the tools needed to make informed decisions regarding their health and safety.

Utilizing social media platforms is another powerful method to reach a wider audience. Campaigns can leverage these platforms to disseminate information quickly and effectively. Engaging posts, infographics, and educational videos can capture attention and encourage sharing among users. Social media can also create a sense of community, where individuals can discuss their concerns and share preventive practices. Regularly updating followers with the latest information and guidelines related to Mpox can help maintain awareness and vigilance.

Collaboration with local healthcare providers can significantly enhance the credibility and reach of awareness campaigns. Healthcare professionals can participate in outreach efforts by sharing their expertise through public forums and health fairs. They can also distribute informational materials, such as brochures and flyers, that outline preventive measures and available resources. By establishing a partnership with trusted medical figures, campaigns can foster trust within the community and encourage individuals to seek medical advice when necessary.

Finally, evaluating the effectiveness of awareness campaigns is essential for continuous improvement. Gathering feedback from participants can provide insights into what information resonated most and what areas may need further emphasis. Analyzing attendance rates, social media engagement, and community feedback will help organizers refine their approaches, ensuring that future campaigns are even more impactful. By prioritizing awareness and education, communities can create a robust defense against the Mpox virus, ultimately contributing to public health and safety.

How To Prevent Mpox Virus

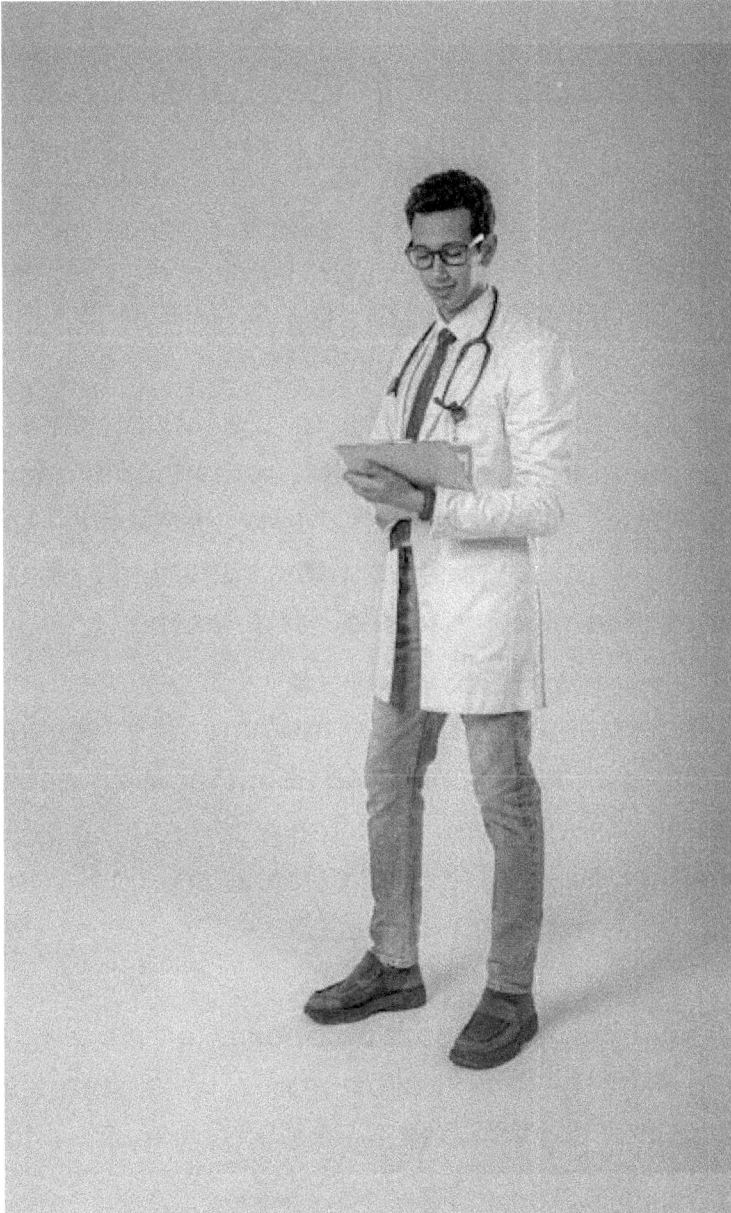

Chapter 6

Responding to Potential Exposure

Recognizing Symptoms

Recognizing symptoms of the Mpox virus is a crucial step in preventing its spread and ensuring timely medical intervention. Mpox, previously known as monkeypox, can present with a variety of symptoms that may resemble those of other illnesses.

Understanding these symptoms is essential for individuals who are concerned about the virus and wish to protect themselves and their communities. Early recognition can lead to quicker isolation and treatment, reducing the risk of transmission.

The initial symptoms of Mpox often include fever, chills, headache, and muscle aches, which can appear within a few days to two weeks after exposure to the virus.

These flu-like symptoms may be accompanied by fatigue and swollen lymph nodes, which is a distinguishing characteristic of Mpox compared to other similar viral infections.

It is vital to monitor these symptoms closely, particularly if you have been in contact with someone diagnosed with Mpox or have traveled to areas where the virus is prevalent.

As the illness progresses, characteristic skin lesions emerge, typically starting as flat lesions that evolve into raised bumps and eventually form pus-filled blisters. These lesions may appear on various parts of the body, including the face, hands, and genital area. The presence of these rashes, especially if accompanied by the flu-like symptoms mentioned earlier, warrants immediate medical attention.

Prompt recognition of these lesions is critical, as they indicate a progression of the disease that requires isolation and treatment to prevent further transmission.

In addition to physical symptoms, individuals should be aware of any unusual changes in their health that could signal an infection. This includes unexplained rashes, particularly if they resemble those associated with Mpox, and any new or worsening flu-like symptoms without an apparent cause. Keeping a detailed record of any potential exposure, travel history, and symptom onset can significantly aid health professionals in making a timely diagnosis and implementing necessary public health measures.

Finally, education and awareness play pivotal roles in recognizing the symptoms of Mpox. Individuals should stay informed about the latest developments regarding the virus, including updates from public health authorities and healthcare providers.

By being proactive and vigilant, those concerned about Mpox can empower themselves and their communities to respond effectively to potential outbreaks, ultimately contributing to public health safety and the prevention of further transmission.

Immediate Steps to Take

In the face of the Mpox virus, immediate action is crucial for individuals concerned about their health and safety. Understanding the virus's transmission methods is the first step. Mpox primarily spreads through close contact with an infected person, particularly via respiratory droplets, skin lesions, or bodily fluids. Recognizing how the virus can be transmitted allows individuals to modify their behaviors and reduce their risk. This includes maintaining distance from those displaying symptoms and avoiding direct contact with rashes or sores that may appear on an infected person's skin.

Personal hygiene is a powerful weapon against the Mpox virus. Regular hand washing with soap and water for at least 20 seconds is essential, especially after being in public spaces or in contact with potentially contaminated surfaces. If soap and water are unavailable, using an alcohol-based hand sanitizer can serve as an effective alternative. Additionally, individuals should avoid touching their face, particularly the eyes, nose, and mouth, with unwashed hands, as this can facilitate the entry of the virus into the body.

Another immediate step to consider is the careful management of one's environment. Keeping living spaces clean and sanitized can significantly mitigate the risk of transmission. Frequently touched surfaces such as doorknobs, light switches, and mobile devices should be cleaned regularly with disinfectants. In communal settings, individuals should be vigilant about their surroundings and encourage others to practice good hygiene. This proactive approach can foster a safer environment for everyone, especially in high-risk areas.

In addition to personal and environmental hygiene, staying informed about Mpox and local outbreaks is vital. Subscribing to health alerts from local health departments or credible organizations can provide timely updates on the virus's status in specific regions.

Understanding the symptoms of Mpox—such as fever, headache, and rash—enables individuals to recognize potential infections early. Prompt identification can lead to quicker isolation and treatment, reducing the risk of spreading the virus to others.

Lastly, vaccination is a critical component of preventing the spread of Mpox. Individuals should consult healthcare providers about the availability of vaccines and their eligibility. Vaccination not only protects the individual but also contributes to community immunity, thereby reducing the overall risk of transmission. Engaging in discussions with healthcare professionals about vaccination options and any concerns can empower individuals to make informed decisions about their health and safety in relation to the Mpox virus. Taking these immediate steps can significantly diminish the risk of infection and promote a safer community environment.

When to Seek Medical Help

When it comes to managing your health in relation to the Mpox virus, understanding when to seek medical help is essential. While many individuals may experience mild symptoms that can be managed at home, there are specific indicators that should prompt immediate medical attention. Recognizing these signs not only ensures personal safety but also contributes to the broader public health effort in controlling potential outbreaks.

One of the primary reasons to consult a healthcare provider is the appearance of symptoms associated with Mpox. These can include fever, fatigue, swollen lymph nodes, and a distinctive rash. If you notice a combination of these symptoms, especially if they worsen over a few days, seeking medical advice is crucial.

Early detection and intervention can significantly affect treatment outcomes and reduce the risk of transmission to others.

In addition to symptomatic concerns, individuals who believe they have been exposed to the Mpox virus are encouraged to reach out to healthcare professionals. Exposure could occur through direct contact with an infected individual or contaminated materials. Even if symptoms are not present, medical professionals can guide you on monitoring your health, conducting tests, or implementing preventive measures to protect yourself and those around you.

Another critical situation that warrants medical attention is the presence of severe symptoms. This includes difficulty breathing, persistent vomiting, or any neurological signs such as confusion or seizures. These symptoms can indicate complications that require immediate care. It is vital to treat such signs seriously, as they could signify a more severe manifestation of the virus or secondary infections that require urgent intervention.

Lastly, it is important to maintain open communication with your healthcare provider about your health history and any underlying conditions that may affect your response to the Mpox virus. Individuals with weakened immune systems or chronic health issues may be at higher risk for severe illness and should remain vigilant. Regular check-ins with medical professionals can provide personalized guidance on risk management, vaccination options, and additional preventive strategies tailored to your specific health needs. Taking proactive steps in collaboration with healthcare providers is a key component of staying safe amid concerns about the Mpox virus.

How To Prevent Mpox Virus

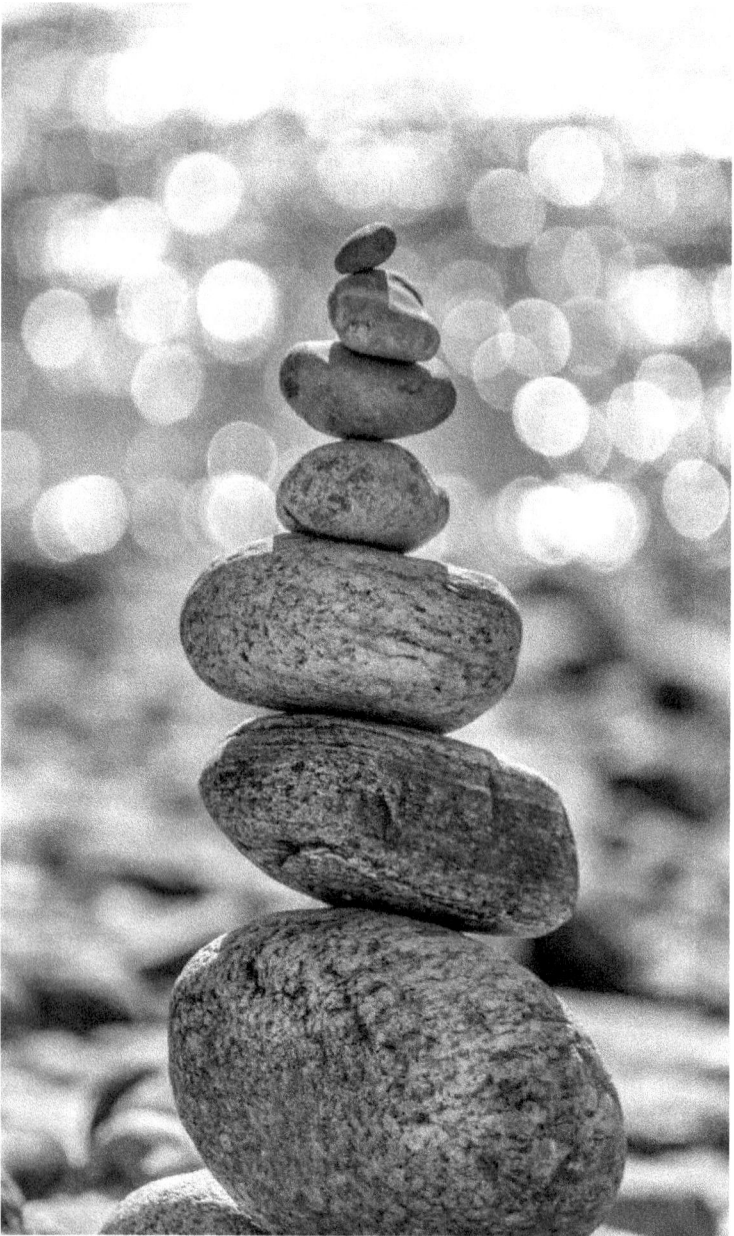

Chapter 7

Mental Health Considerations

Coping with Anxiety and Fear

Coping with anxiety and fear is an essential aspect of managing the emotional toll that the Mpox virus can exert on individuals and communities. The uncertainty surrounding an outbreak can lead to heightened anxiety levels, especially among those who are particularly vulnerable or have a close connection to affected individuals.

Understanding the nature of these feelings and employing effective coping strategies can help mitigate anxiety and foster a sense of control during uncertain times. By acknowledging these emotions, individuals can take proactive steps to safeguard their mental health while remaining informed and vigilant.

One of the primary ways to cope with anxiety is to stay informed through reliable sources. Misinformation can exacerbate fears and lead to unnecessary panic. It is crucial to rely on trusted health organizations, such as the Centers for Disease Control and Prevention (CDC) and the World Health Organization (WHO), for accurate updates on the Mpox virus. By understanding the transmission methods, symptoms, and preventive measures, individuals can feel more empowered and less overwhelmed. Furthermore, being informed allows individuals to separate fact from fiction, reducing the anxiety that often stems from uncertainty.

Developing a structured routine can also be beneficial in managing anxiety related to the Mpox virus. Establishing a daily schedule that includes time for work, self-care, and relaxation can create a sense of normalcy amidst the chaos. Incorporating activities that promote mental well-being, such as exercise, mindfulness, or hobbies, can provide an effective outlet for stress. Engaging in regular physical activity has been shown to reduce anxiety and improve mood, while mindfulness practices like meditation can enhance emotional regulation and resilience.

Connecting with others is another vital aspect of coping with anxiety and fear. Sharing feelings and experiences with friends, family, or support groups can foster a sense of community and remind individuals that they are not alone in their concerns. Open conversations about fears related to the Mpox virus can help normalize these feelings and reduce stigma. Additionally, seeking support from mental health professionals may be beneficial for those who find their anxiety overwhelming or persistent. Professional guidance can provide individuals with tailored coping strategies and resources to navigate their fears effectively.

Lastly, it is important to practice self-compassion during times of heightened anxiety. Recognizing that it is natural to feel anxious in response to a public health crisis allows individuals to be kinder to themselves. Self-care practices, such as ensuring adequate sleep, maintaining a healthy diet, and engaging in enjoyable activities, are essential for emotional well-being. By prioritizing self-care and understanding that anxiety is a common response to fear, individuals can cultivate resilience and better manage their concerns about the Mpox virus.

Support Systems and Resources

In the face of the Mpox virus, having access to effective support systems and resources is crucial for individuals concerned about prevention. These systems encompass a variety of entities, including healthcare providers, community organizations, and digital platforms dedicated to disseminating accurate information. Understanding how to leverage these resources can empower individuals to take proactive measures in safeguarding their health and the health of those around them.

Healthcare providers play a pivotal role in offering guidance and support. They are often the first point of contact for individuals seeking information about Mpox and its prevention. Regular consultations with healthcare professionals can lead to personalized advice based on an individual's health history and lifestyle. Moreover, healthcare providers can facilitate access to vaccinations and preventive treatments, significantly reducing the risk of infection. Building a trusting relationship with medical professionals can enhance the effectiveness of preventive strategies, as they can offer tailored recommendations and ongoing monitoring.

Community organizations are invaluable in fostering awareness and providing resources related to Mpox prevention. Many local health departments and non-profit organizations conduct outreach programs aimed at educating the public about the virus and its transmission.

These organizations often host workshops, distribute informational materials, and create campaigns to encourage safe practices. Engaging with these community resources not only increases knowledge but also fosters a sense of solidarity among individuals concerned about Mpox. Such community involvement can lead to collective action, which is essential in combating the spread of the virus.

Digital platforms serve as another critical component of support systems for those seeking to prevent Mpox. Numerous websites, social media channels, and mobile applications are dedicated to providing up-to-date information on the virus. These digital resources can offer real-time updates on outbreaks, vaccination availability, and preventive measures.

Additionally, online forums and support groups can create a space for individuals to share experiences, ask questions, and receive encouragement from others who share similar concerns. Utilizing these platforms can enhance understanding and foster a community of informed individuals committed to prevention.

Lastly, educational institutions also play a significant role in disseminating information about Mpox. Schools and universities can implement programs that educate students and staff on the importance of hygiene practices, vaccination, and recognizing the symptoms of Mpox.

By integrating this information into health curricula or hosting seminars, educational institutions can equip individuals with the knowledge needed to protect themselves and others. Collaboration between educational bodies, healthcare professionals, and community organizations can create a comprehensive approach to prevention, ensuring that accurate information reaches a broad audience.

In summary, an effective support system for preventing Mpox includes healthcare providers, community organizations, digital platforms, and educational institutions. By tapping into these resources, individuals can enhance their understanding of the virus, adopt preventive measures, and contribute to a collective effort in safeguarding public health. Empowerment through knowledge and community support is essential in the ongoing fight against Mpox.

Promoting Resilience

Promoting resilience in the face of the Mpox virus involves empowering individuals and communities with the knowledge and tools necessary to mitigate risks and enhance well-being.

Resilience, in this context, is the ability to adapt to challenges posed by infectious diseases, maintaining mental and physical health while taking proactive steps to minimize exposure. By fostering a culture of preparedness and awareness, individuals can significantly reduce their vulnerability to Mpox and similar health threats.

Education is the cornerstone of resilience. Understanding how the Mpox virus spreads, its symptoms, and the populations at higher risk is crucial for effective prevention. Individuals should familiarize themselves with the transmission routes, which include close physical contact with infected individuals or contaminated objects.

Public health campaigns play a vital role in disseminating this information, encouraging people to stay informed through reputable sources such as the World Health Organization (WHO) and the Centers for Disease Control and Prevention (CDC). Knowledge empowers individuals to recognize potential risks and take appropriate action to protect themselves and their communities.

Behavioral changes are essential in promoting resilience against the Mpox virus. Practicing good hygiene, such as regular handwashing with soap and water or using hand sanitizer, can greatly reduce the risk of transmission. Additionally, maintaining physical distance in crowded settings and avoiding close contact with those who display symptoms of the virus are effective strategies.

Encouraging these habits within communities fosters a collective sense of responsibility, where each person's actions contribute to the overall safety and health of the group. The more ingrained these practices become, the more resilient communities will be in the face of outbreaks.

Mental resilience is equally important in combating the stress and anxiety that can arise during health crises like an Mpox outbreak. Communities should prioritize mental health resources and support systems, providing access to counseling and stress management techniques.

Open discussions about fears and concerns can help individuals process their emotions, reducing feelings of isolation and helplessness. Furthermore, fostering strong social connections can enhance resilience, as individuals who feel supported are more likely to engage in preventive behaviors and seek help when needed.

In conclusion, promoting resilience against the Mpox virus requires a multifaceted approach that encompasses education, behavioral change, and mental health support. By equipping individuals with the necessary tools and knowledge, communities can enhance their overall preparedness and capacity to respond to health threats.

This proactive approach not only reduces the risk of infection but also strengthens the social fabric, enabling communities to thrive even in challenging circumstances. Through collective efforts, resilience can be cultivated, ensuring that individuals are better prepared to face the uncertainties of infectious diseases like Mpox.

How To Prevent Mpox Virus

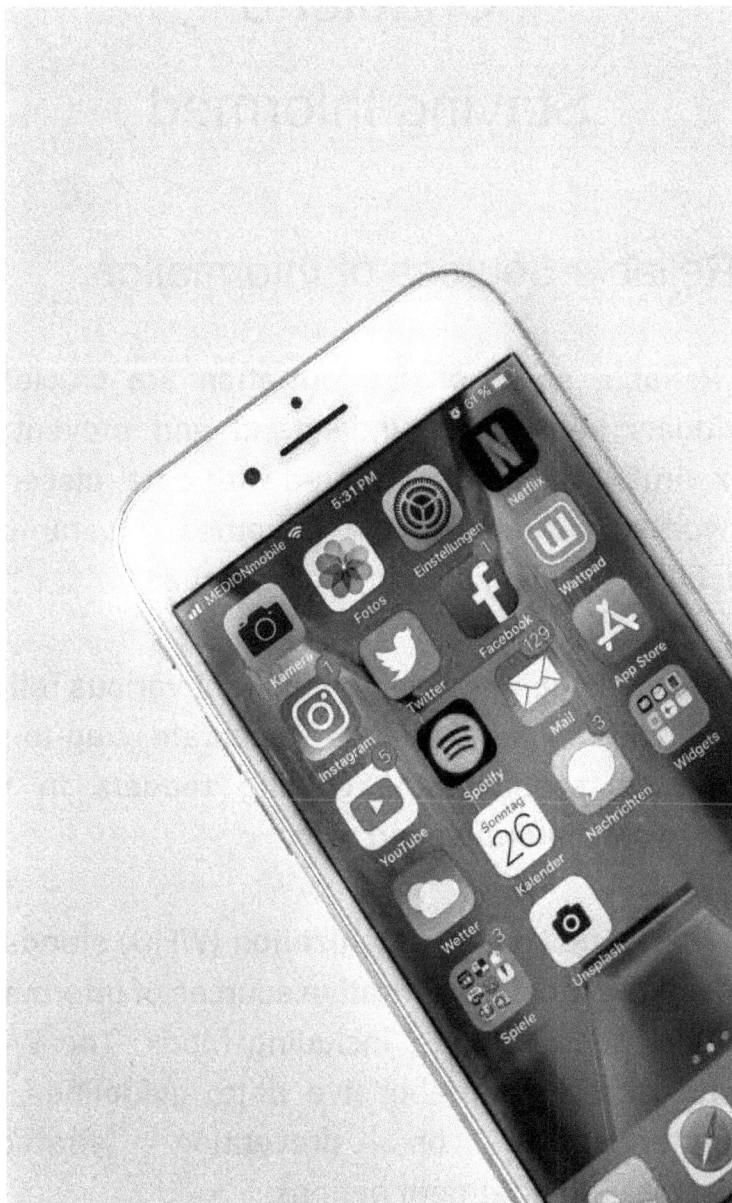

Chapter 8

Staying Informed

Reliable Sources of Information

Reliable sources of information are crucial for individuals seeking to understand and prevent the Mpox virus. In a world saturated with data, discerning trustworthy information becomes paramount, especially regarding health-related issues.

This subchapter aims to highlight various reliable sources that can provide accurate, up-to-date information about Mpox, guiding readers in their efforts to stay informed and safe.

The World Health Organization (WHO) stands out as one of the most authoritative sources of information on global health issues, including Mpox. The WHO's website offers comprehensive data, guidelines, and recommendations on prevention strategies, symptoms, and treatment options.

By consulting the WHO, individuals can access the latest research findings and public health advice, ensuring they remain well-informed about the evolving nature of the Mpox virus and its implications for public health.

In addition to the WHO, the Centers for Disease Control and Prevention (CDC) serves as another vital resource for individuals concerned about Mpox. The CDC provides detailed information on transmission methods, risk factors, and preventive measures specific to the virus.

Their guidelines are especially useful for individuals in high-risk environments or those who may have been exposed to the virus. By relying on the CDC's insights, readers can develop a clearer understanding of how to protect themselves and their communities.

Local health departments also play a significant role in disseminating information about Mpox. These agencies often tailor their advice to the specific needs of their communities, addressing local outbreaks and providing resources for testing and vaccination.

Individuals should actively engage with their local health departments, attending community meetings or following their social media channels for real-time updates and recommendations. This localized approach ensures that the information is relevant and actionable, enhancing community resilience against the virus.

Lastly, peer-reviewed journals and academic institutions contribute valuable knowledge regarding the Mpox virus. Research studies published in reputable journals offer in-depth analyses of the virus's characteristics, transmission dynamics, and effective prevention strategies.

Engaging with this literature can empower individuals with the scientific understanding necessary to navigate discussions and make informed decisions about their health. By combining insights from these reliable sources, readers can build a well-rounded perspective on Mpox prevention, leading to safer practices and greater community awareness.

Monitoring Updates and Guidelines

Monitoring updates and guidelines related to the Mpox virus is essential for anyone concerned about their health and safety. As the situation surrounding infectious diseases can evolve rapidly, staying informed is crucial in preventing transmission and protecting oneself and the community. This subchapter outlines the importance of regularly checking credible sources for updates, understanding the guidelines provided by health authorities, and adapting personal practices accordingly.

Health organizations, such as the World Health Organization (WHO) and the Centers for Disease Control and Prevention (CDC), are primary sources for the latest information regarding Mpox. These organizations frequently update their guidelines based on new scientific evidence and epidemiological data. It is vital for individuals to follow these updates closely to understand the current risk levels, vaccination availability, and changes in recommended preventive measures. Subscribing to newsletters or alerts from these organizations can facilitate timely access to crucial information.

Local health departments also play a significant role in disseminating information about Mpox within specific communities. They provide tailored guidance based on regional outbreaks and public health assessments. Engaging with local health initiatives can inform individuals about vaccination clinics, awareness campaigns, and community education efforts.

By participating in local health events or forums, individuals can gain insights into how the community is responding to the Mpox virus and how they can contribute to those efforts.

In addition to monitoring official sources, it is beneficial to remain aware of emerging research and news regarding Mpox. Scientific journals, reputable news outlets, and public health blogs can provide valuable insights into the virus's transmission dynamics, symptomatology, and treatment options. Staying updated on these developments can help individuals make informed decisions about their health, recognize symptoms early, and seek medical advice when necessary.

Finally, adapting personal hygiene and preventive practices in response to new guidelines is critical. As updates are released, individuals should be prepared to modify their behaviors, such as increasing social distancing, wearing masks in crowded settings, or enhancing hand hygiene practices. This proactive approach not only protects individual health but also contributes to broader community safety by reducing the potential spread of the virus. By staying informed and adaptable, individuals can significantly mitigate their risk of Mpox infection.

Importance of Continuous Learning

Continuous learning plays a crucial role in effectively preventing the Mpox virus. As the world grapples with emerging infectious diseases, the information landscape is constantly evolving. New research findings, treatment protocols, and preventive measures are regularly introduced, making it essential for individuals concerned about their health and safety to stay informed. Continuous learning empowers individuals to understand the nature of the Mpox virus, recognize its transmission routes, and implement effective preventive strategies.

One of the primary reasons continuous learning is important in the context of Mpox is the dynamic nature of viral outbreaks. The Mpox virus, like many other pathogens, can mutate and adapt, which may influence its transmissibility and severity. By engaging in ongoing education, individuals can keep abreast of the latest findings related to the virus, including potential changes in its behavior and epidemiology. This knowledge is vital for making informed decisions about personal safety measures and community health practices.

Moreover, continuous learning fosters critical thinking and encourages an adaptive mindset. As new information emerges about Mpox, individuals may encounter conflicting advice or recommendations. A commitment to lifelong learning equips individuals with the skills to evaluate sources, discern credible information, and differentiate between fact and misinformation.

This critical approach is especially important in the age of social media, where misleading information can spread rapidly and influence public perception and behavior regarding health risks.

In addition to enhancing personal knowledge, continuous learning also contributes to community resilience against the Mpox virus. When individuals actively seek to educate themselves and share their knowledge with others, they create a ripple effect that strengthens community awareness and preparedness.

Community members who understand the importance of vaccination, hygiene practices, and early symptom recognition can collectively reduce the virus's spread. Collaborative learning initiatives, such as workshops and discussions, can further empower communities to develop effective strategies for prevention.

Lastly, committing to continuous learning about Mpox not only benefits personal health but also contributes to global efforts in combating infectious diseases. By understanding the factors that facilitate outbreaks and the best practices for prevention, individuals can participate in broader public health initiatives and advocacy. This engagement can lead to better policies, increased funding for research, and improved healthcare responses to outbreaks.

In a world where infectious diseases are a persistent threat, the importance of continuous learning cannot be overstated; it is an essential tool for safeguarding both individual and public health.

How To Prevent Mpox Virus

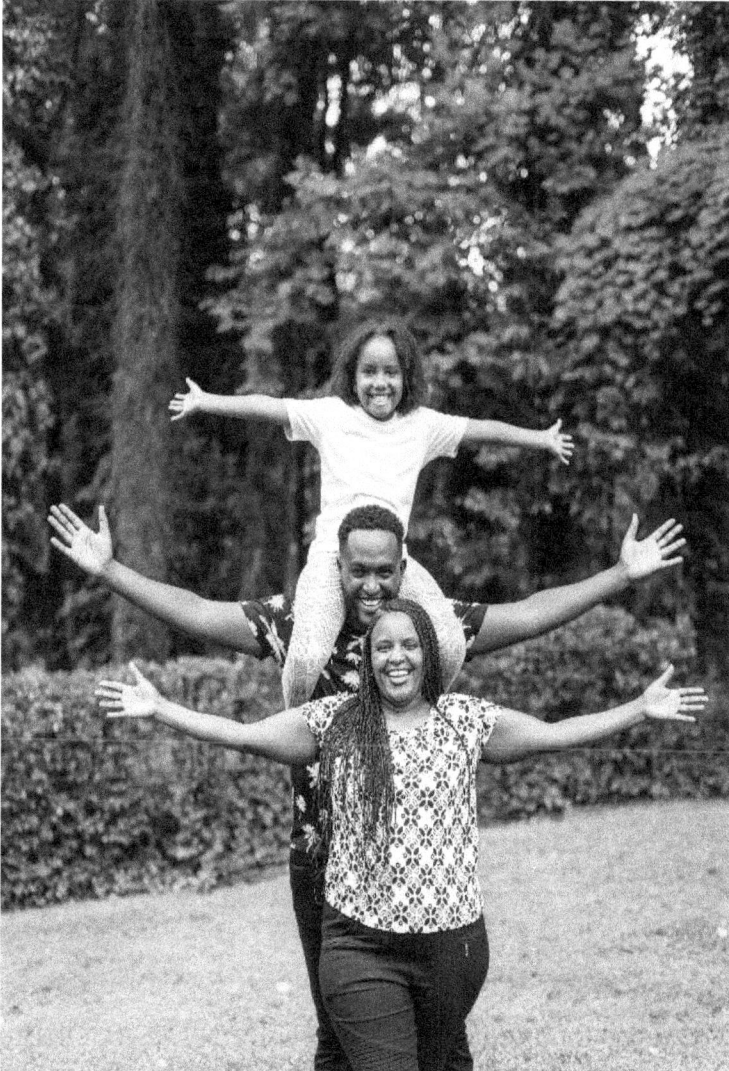

Chapter 9

Personal Action Plans

Creating a Personal Safety Plan

Creating a Personal Safety Plan is an essential step for individuals concerned about the Mpox virus. This virus, which can pose significant health risks, has raised awareness about the importance of personal health strategies. A well-structured safety plan not only equips you with the knowledge to protect yourself but also empowers you to act decisively in various situations. This plan should encompass awareness, prevention, and response strategies tailored to your lifestyle and environment.

The first step in developing a personal safety plan is to stay informed about the Mpox virus. Understanding its transmission, symptoms, and potential complications is crucial. The virus primarily spreads through close contact with infected individuals or contaminated surfaces.

Educate yourself on the various modes of transmission, including physical touch, respiratory droplets, and shared items.

Reliable resources, such as the Centers for Disease Control and Prevention (CDC) and local health departments, provide valuable information that can help you identify risks and implement preventative measures effectively.

Next, consider your daily routines and identify areas where you can minimize exposure to the virus. This might involve altering social habits, such as avoiding crowded places or refraining from physical contact during gatherings. In addition, practicing good hygiene is paramount. Wash your hands frequently with soap and water for at least 20 seconds, or use hand sanitizer with at least 60% alcohol when soap is unavailable.

Make it a habit to clean and disinfect frequently touched surfaces in your home, workplace, and any shared spaces to further reduce the risk of viral transmission.

Incorporating health monitoring into your personal safety plan is also vital. Keep track of your health and any symptoms that may arise. If you experience signs consistent with the Mpox virus, such as fever, rash, or swollen lymph nodes, seek medical advice immediately. Additionally, staying connected with your healthcare provider can help you access preventative resources, such as vaccinations or post-exposure prophylaxis, if necessary. Maintaining open communication with friends and family about your safety plan can also foster a supportive environment, encouraging collective responsibility for health.

Lastly, prepare for potential scenarios where you may encounter the virus. This includes having a plan in place for self-isolation if you or someone in your household becomes infected. Ensure you have supplies on hand, such as medications, food, and hygiene products, to minimize the need for outside contact during isolation. Familiarize yourself with local health resources and support networks that can assist you in case of an outbreak. By proactively addressing these potential challenges, you can further enhance your personal safety plan, ensuring that you and your loved ones are well-equipped to navigate the risks associated with the Mpox virus.

Family Safety Strategies

In the face of the Mpox virus, prioritizing the safety of your family is essential. The Mpox virus, previously known as monkeypox, is a viral zoonotic disease that can spread through close contact with infected individuals or animals. To protect your loved ones, implementing effective safety strategies is crucial. These strategies not only focus on prevention but also aim to enhance awareness and preparedness within the family unit.

One of the most effective strategies is education. Families should stay informed about the Mpox virus, its modes of transmission, and its symptoms. Regularly discussing these topics can help demystify the virus and reduce fear. Parents can utilize age-appropriate resources, such as books or engaging online materials, to explain the virus to children.

Understanding the importance of hygiene practices, such as regular handwashing and avoiding close contact with symptomatic individuals, can empower family members to take responsibility for their health.

Establishing a hygiene routine is another critical component of family safety. This can include regular handwashing with soap and water, the use of hand sanitizers with at least 60% alcohol, and ensuring that household surfaces are routinely cleaned and disinfected. Families should create a checklist of hygiene practices to reinforce these habits. Additionally, teaching children the importance of not sharing personal items, such as towels or utensils, can further minimize the risk of transmission within the home.

In the event of a suspected exposure, having an action plan is vital. Families should be prepared to identify symptoms of Mpox and know when to seek medical attention. Establishing a communication plan that includes emergency contacts and a designated healthcare provider can streamline responses during a crisis.

Keeping a well-stocked first aid kit and ensuring that family members are familiar with its contents can also provide peace of mind. Regularly reviewing this plan ensures that everyone knows their role in safeguarding the family's health.

Lastly, promoting a supportive environment can significantly enhance family safety. Open communication about health concerns, fears, and experiences can foster resilience and cooperation among family members. In times of heightened anxiety regarding the Mpox virus, providing emotional support is just as important as physical safety. Engaging in family activities that promote well-being, such as exercise or mindfulness practices, can help alleviate stress and reinforce the importance of staying healthy together. By adopting these family safety strategies, you can create a strong foundation for preventing the Mpox virus and ensuring the well-being of your loved ones.

Workplace Preparedness

Workplace preparedness is a critical component in the fight against the Mpox virus. Given the virus's potential for transmission in communal settings, employers and employees alike must adopt proactive measures to mitigate risks. This subchapter will outline essential strategies that organizations can implement to ensure a safe and healthy work environment, ultimately contributing to the broader public health efforts against the Mpox virus.

First and foremost, establishing clear communication channels is vital. Organizations should disseminate information regarding the Mpox virus, including symptoms, transmission methods, and preventive measures. Regular updates and training sessions can bolster employee awareness and foster a culture of safety. Employers can utilize newsletters, emails, and team meetings to reinforce the importance of vigilance and encourage open discussions about any concerns related to workplace health.

In addition to education, implementing robust hygiene protocols is essential. Workplaces should provide adequate handwashing facilities and ensure that hand sanitizers are readily available throughout the premises.

Frequent cleaning and disinfection of commonly touched surfaces—such as doorknobs, light switches, and shared equipment—should be prioritized. These routines not only reduce the risk of the virus spreading but also promote a general atmosphere of cleanliness and care within the workplace.

Another crucial aspect of workplace preparedness is the development of a response plan in the event of a suspected Mpox case. This plan should outline steps for isolating the individual, notifying health authorities, and conducting contact tracing. Having a clear protocol in place ensures that all employees know how to act swiftly and effectively, minimizing potential exposure and safeguarding the health of the entire workforce. Regular drills and simulations can help familiarize staff with these procedures, reinforcing their importance.

Lastly, fostering a supportive work environment can greatly enhance workplace preparedness. Employers should encourage employees to report any symptoms or health concerns without fear of reprisal. Implementing flexible sick leave policies can ensure that individuals feel comfortable staying home if they are unwell, thereby reducing the risk of spreading the virus.

Additionally, promoting mental health resources and wellness programs can help employees cope with the stress and anxiety that may arise during outbreaks, ultimately contributing to a more resilient workforce.

In conclusion, workplace preparedness against the Mpox virus requires a multifaceted approach that includes clear communication, strict hygiene practices, effective response plans, and a supportive environment. By prioritizing these strategies, organizations can not only protect their employees but also play a vital role in the broader public health initiative to prevent the spread of Mpox. As the understanding of this virus evolves, continuous evaluation and adaptation of workplace protocols will be necessary to ensure ongoing safety and preparedness.

How To Prevent Mpox Virus

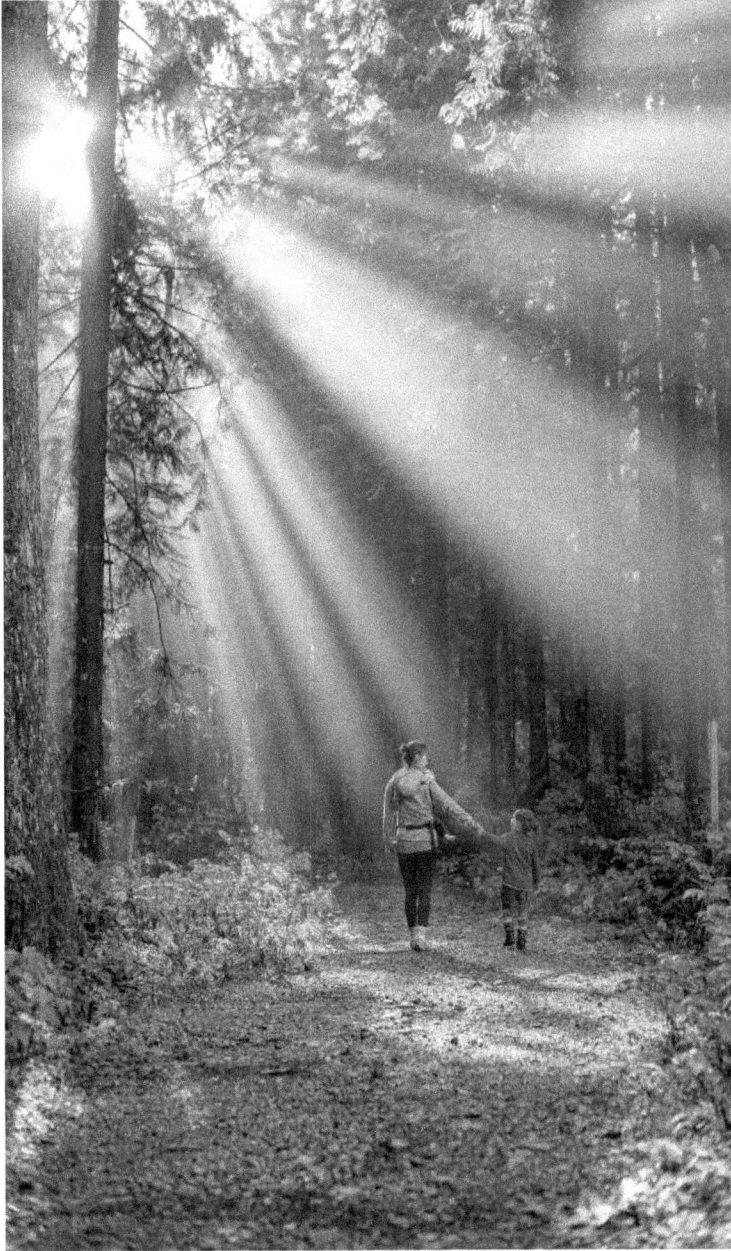

Chapter 10

Future Considerations

Ongoing Research and Developments

Ongoing research and developments in the field of mpox virus prevention are crucial for understanding and mitigating its spread. Scientists and public health officials are actively engaged in studying the virus's transmission dynamics, its genetic variations, and the efficacy of current preventive measures.

This research is vital not only for developing targeted interventions but also for informing the public about how to stay safe. Understanding the latest findings can empower individuals to adopt better practices in their daily lives, reducing the risk of infection.

One of the key areas of focus in current research is the exploration of vaccines specifically designed to combat the mpox virus. While traditional vaccination strategies have been effective for other viral infections, scientists are investigating how to create a vaccine that offers robust and lasting protection against mpox. Clinical trials are ongoing to evaluate the safety and effectiveness of these vaccines, with preliminary results suggesting promising immune responses. As these studies progress, they hold the potential to provide a significant tool in the public health arsenal against mpox.

In addition to vaccine development, researchers are examining the role of antiviral treatments in managing mpox infections. Preliminary studies are assessing various antiviral drugs and their efficacy in reducing the viral load and severity of symptoms in infected individuals. This research is particularly important for individuals at higher risk of severe disease outcomes, such as those with compromised immune systems. The findings from these studies could lead to the establishment of treatment protocols that not only aid in recovery but also help prevent further transmission in community settings.

Public health campaigns are also evolving as new research sheds light on the most effective communication strategies to educate communities about mpox. Ongoing studies are analyzing the impact of various messaging approaches to ensure that information is accessible and resonates with diverse populations. This is particularly pertinent in marginalized communities, where misinformation can hinder prevention efforts.

By tailoring campaigns to address specific cultural and societal contexts, public health officials aim to improve awareness and encourage safer behaviors that reduce the risk of mpox transmission.

Finally, collaboration between international health organizations, governments, and research institutions is essential to address the global nature of mpox. Ongoing developments in surveillance systems and data sharing are crucial for tracking outbreaks and understanding the virus's epidemiology. This collaborative approach not only enhances the ability to respond to current outbreaks but also equips health authorities with the knowledge needed to prevent future occurrences.

As research continues to evolve, staying informed about the latest developments will help individuals make educated decisions to protect themselves and their communities from the mpox virus.

The Role of Public Health Policy

Public health policy plays a crucial role in the prevention and control of infectious diseases, including the Mpox virus. These policies are designed to protect populations by establishing guidelines and regulations that promote health and safety. Understanding the significance of public health policy can empower individuals and communities to take proactive measures against the spread of Mpox.

This subchapter will explore the key components of public health policy related to Mpox, the importance of community engagement, and the impact of these policies on individual behaviors.

One of the primary functions of public health policy is the development of surveillance systems that monitor the incidence and prevalence of diseases like Mpox. These systems are essential for identifying outbreaks early, allowing public health officials to respond swiftly.

Timely data collection and analysis enable health authorities to track the virus's spread, assess risk factors, and allocate resources effectively. This proactive approach not only helps in managing current outbreaks but also prepares communities for potential future threats, fostering a culture of preparedness and responsiveness.

Public health policy also encompasses vaccination programs, which are critical in preventing the transmission of Mpox. Vaccines have proven effective in controlling various infectious diseases, and their inclusion in public health strategies significantly reduces the risk of widespread outbreaks. Health authorities must prioritize access to vaccines, particularly for high-risk populations, and implement educational campaigns to inform the public about the benefits of vaccination.

By addressing misconceptions and providing clear information, public health policies can enhance community uptake of vaccines, ultimately safeguarding public health.

Another vital aspect of public health policy is the promotion of health education and awareness initiatives. These programs aim to inform individuals about the Mpox virus, its transmission methods, and preventive measures. Effective communication strategies are essential to ensure that the public understands how to reduce their risk of exposure.

By providing accessible information through various channels—such as social media, community workshops, and healthcare providers—public health policies can empower individuals to make informed choices regarding their health and safety. This education is particularly important in dispelling stigma associated with the virus, fostering a more supportive environment for those affected.

Finally, public health policy relies on collaboration among various stakeholders, including government agencies, healthcare providers, non-profit organizations, and the community. This multi-faceted approach ensures that prevention strategies are comprehensive and inclusive. Engaging community members in the decision-making process fosters trust and encourages participation in health initiatives. By recognizing the unique needs and concerns of different populations, public health policies can be tailored to address specific challenges related to Mpox prevention. Effective collaboration not only enhances the implementation of policies but also strengthens community resilience against infectious diseases, ensuring a safer environment for all.

Long-term Strategies for Prevention

Long-term strategies for preventing Mpox virus are essential for individuals and communities concerned about this emerging health threat. As public awareness grows, it becomes increasingly important to understand how to implement effective prevention measures that can reduce the risk of infection over time.

This subchapter outlines several critical approaches that can be adopted on both personal and community levels to mitigate the impact of Mpox virus.

One of the most important long-term strategies for preventing Mpox is fostering a culture of health education. This involves not only increasing awareness about the virus but also promoting knowledge about its transmission and symptoms. Educational programs should be designed for various demographics, including schools, workplaces, and community centers.

By providing accessible information and resources, individuals can make informed decisions about their health and take proactive steps to protect themselves and others. Workshops, seminars, and informational campaigns can play a vital role in dispelling myths and addressing misconceptions about Mpox.

Vaccination is another cornerstone of long-term prevention strategies. While vaccines for Mpox may not be universally available, encouraging vaccination against related viruses can help bolster community immunity. Public health authorities should advocate for research and the development of effective vaccines specifically targeting Mpox.

Additionally, individuals should stay informed about vaccination recommendations and participate in any available vaccination programs. A collective commitment to vaccination can significantly decrease the spread of the virus and protect vulnerable populations.

Behavioral changes are crucial in preventing Mpox transmission over the long term. Individuals should be encouraged to adopt safer practices, particularly in social settings where the virus may spread more easily. This includes regular handwashing, maintaining personal hygiene, and practicing safe sex.

Moreover, promoting the use of personal protective equipment (PPE) in high-risk environments, such as healthcare facilities and crowded gatherings, can further reduce the chances of infection. Community outreach programs can help normalize these practices, making them a part of everyday life.

Building strong community networks is also vital for long-term prevention strategies. Collaborative efforts among local organizations, healthcare providers, and public health officials can create a robust support system for monitoring and addressing Mpox outbreaks. This can involve establishing communication channels for sharing information about risk factors, symptoms, and preventive measures.

Engaging community leaders and influencers can help disseminate important health messages more effectively, ensuring that prevention strategies reach diverse populations.

Lastly, ongoing research and surveillance are critical components of a comprehensive prevention strategy. Advocating for funding and resources to support studies on Mpox virus transmission, immunity, and treatment options will enhance our understanding of the virus and inform public health strategies. Surveillance systems need to be in place to track the incidence of Mpox cases and identify potential outbreaks early.

By prioritizing research and data collection, communities can remain vigilant and responsive, adapting their prevention strategies as new information becomes available. Together, these long-term strategies will empower individuals and communities to stay safe and reduce the risk of Mpox virus transmission.

Author Notes & Acknowledgments

First and foremost, I would like to express my deepest gratitude to the people who inspired and supported me throughout the journey of writing this book. This project would not have been possible without their unwavering belief in me and their invaluable contributions.

To my wife, thank you for your constant encouragement and understanding. Your love and support have been my anchor during the challenging times of researching and writing this book. Your belief in my ability to make a difference in people's lives has been my driving force.

I would also like to disclose that this book contains some renewed artificial intelligence-generated content. I really appreciate very recent technological innovation by outstanding scientists and of course our reader's understanding.

Lastly, I want to express my deepest gratitude to the readers of this book. I sincerely hope the strategies and methods outlined within these pages will provide you with the knowledge and tools needed to truly make your life much better. Your commitment to seeking any good solutions and willingness to explore multiple methods is commendable.

Author Bio

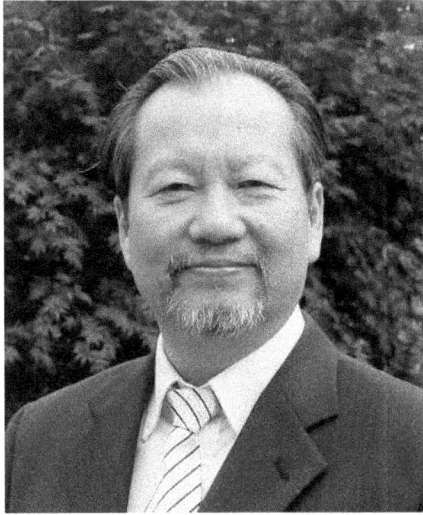

Johnson Wu earned his MD in 1982. With over 40 years of clinical experience, he has worked in hospitals in Zhejiang and Shanghai, China, as well as the Royal Marsden Hospital (part of Imperial College) in London, UK.

Upon the recommendation of Sir Aaron Klug, the president of The Royal Society and a Nobel Prize winner in Chemistry, Dr. Wu was honorably awarded a British Royal Society Fellowship. He has published medical books and articles in seven countries and currently practices medicine in Canada.

www.ingramcontent.com/pod-product-compliance
Lightning Source LLC
Chambersburg PA
CBHW060250030426
42335CB00014B/1645